I0095827

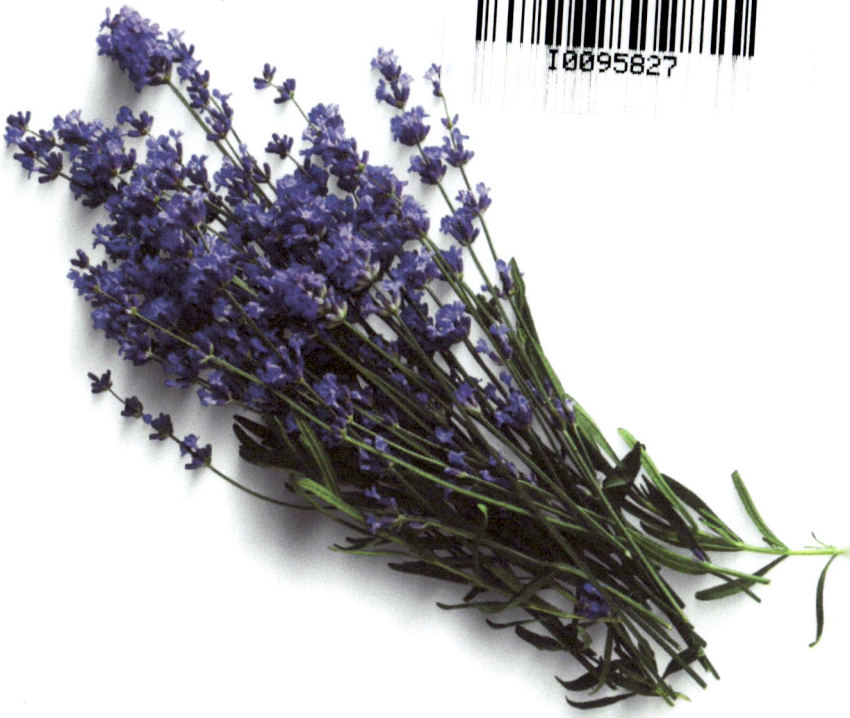

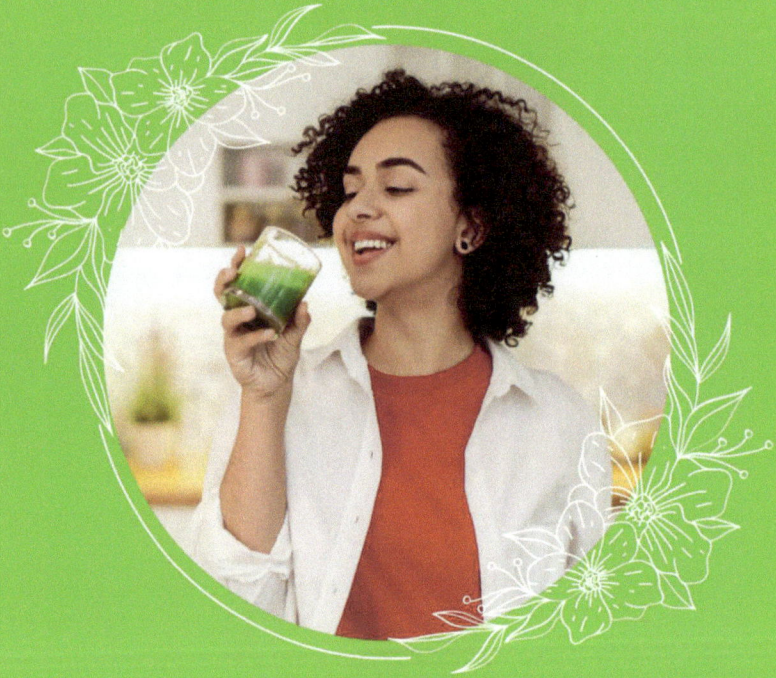

# 21-Day
# Cleanse Meal Plan:
## Supporting Mental
## Health and Detox

# Introduction

Welcome to the 21-Day Mind-Body Detox with Fuller Cleanze Detox Tea, an immersive program designed to bring balance, vitality, and clarity to your body and mind. Created by Dr. Arleen A. Fuller, PhD, this program draws on her extensive experience in natural health and holistic wellness.

Dr. Fuller has dedicated her life to helping people cleanse their bodies and rejuvenate their minds through a science-based approach to natural detoxification, mental clarity, and physical wellness. With a deep commitment to harnessing the power of nature, she developed the Fuller Cleanze Detox Tea—an herbal blend designed to complement this journey by using the natural cleansing powers of dandelion root, hyssop, and lavender.

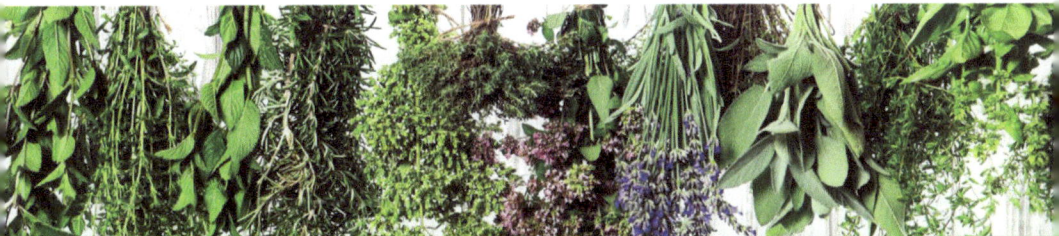

In crafting this book, Dr. Fuller sought to provide a comprehensive, supportive experience that is easy to follow and impactful. With the assistance of AI technology, we've tailored this guide to include a variety of detox-friendly foods, delicious meal plans, and reflective journaling prompts, offering an accessible, adaptable path to wellness. The AI-supported structure ensures that you have substitution options for each day, allowing you to personalize your cleanse experience while staying within the program's beneficial framework.

# Fuller Cleanze Detox Tea: A Natural Detox for Body and Mind

## Ingredients

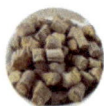

**Dandelion Root:** Known for supporting liver health and detoxification, dandelion root helps the body process and eliminate toxins more efficiently. Its anti-inflammatory properties also aid digestion, which is often linked to improved mood and energy levels.

**Hyssop:** Traditionally used to relieve digestive issues and respiratory ailments, hyssop promotes calmness and is known for its mildly sedative effect, helping reduce anxiety and support relaxation.

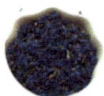

**Lavender:** Often used to alleviate stress and promote calm, lavender can help manage anxiety and improve sleep quality, directly benefiting mental health by calming the nervous system.

Together, these herbs in Fuller Cleanze Detox Tea provide a holistic approach to detoxing by cleansing the body while calming the mind. When enjoyed regularly, the tea can improve digestion, reduce bloating, support liver health, and provide a sense of tranquility, especially when consumed as part of a mindful daily routine.

# 21-Day Cleanze Meal Plan

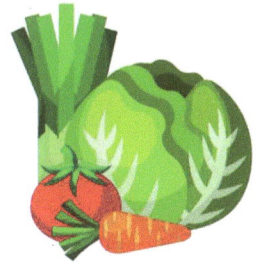

The 21-day meal plan enhances the tea's effects by incorporating foods rich in nutrients that promote physical detox and emotional well-being:

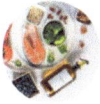

**Nutrient-Dense Foods for Stable Energy:** Whole foods like leafy greens, berries, nuts, seeds, lean proteins, and complex carbs (quinoa, sweet potatoes) help maintain stable blood sugar levels. Balanced blood sugar prevents mood swings, providing a steady supply of energy that supports both physical and mental stamina.

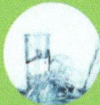

**Hydration:** Staying hydrated is crucial for optimal brain function. Water and hydrating foods (cucumbers, melons) included in the plan, along with Fuller Cleanze Tea, help flush out toxins while supporting cognitive focus and mood stability.

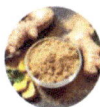

**Anti-Inflammatory Ingredients:** Many foods in this plan, such as turmeric, ginger, and leafy greens, have anti-inflammatory properties. Chronic inflammation is linked to mental health issues like depression and anxiety, so including anti-inflammatory foods can support a more balanced mental state.

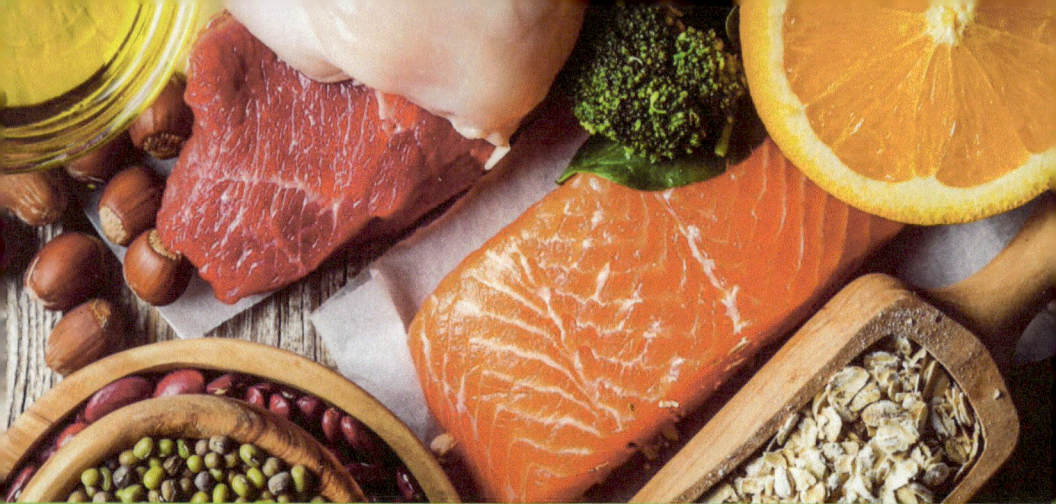

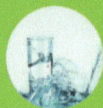

**Promoting Serotonin Production:** Foods high in fiber (oats, brown rice, beans) and omega-3 fatty acids (salmon, walnuts) contribute to gut health. Since a large portion of serotonin (the "feel-good" hormone) is produced in the gut, a healthy digestive system can support better mood regulation and reduce stress.

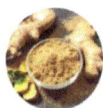

**Relaxing Evening Routine:** Each day concludes with herbal tea like dandelion, ginger, or chamomile. This routine, combined with the Fuller Cleanze Detox Tea, fosters relaxation and sets the stage for a good night's sleep, which is crucial for mental clarity, emotional resilience, and stress reduction.

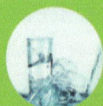

**Mindful Eating and Self-Care:** The cleanse encourages mindful eating and self-care habits like deep breathing, light exercise, and journaling, all of which are beneficial for managing stress, reducing anxiety, and improving focus.

# Mental Health Benefits of the Cleanse

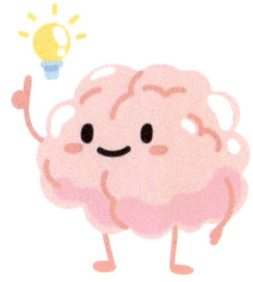

The Fuller Cleanze Detox Tea, combined with the cleanse's nutrient-rich foods, hydration, and relaxation habits, directly supports mental health by:

- **Reducing Anxiety and Stress:** Lavender and hyssop in the tea, along with magnesium-rich foods (leafy greens, nuts), promote relaxation, helping to alleviate anxiety and tension.

- **Improving Sleep Quality:** The calming effects of lavender tea before bed help regulate the sleep cycle, which is essential for emotional balance and mental clarity.

- **Enhancing Mood Stability:** Nutrient-dense meals prevent energy crashes, while foods supporting gut health (probiotic-rich ingredients, fiber, and omega-3s) boost serotonin, enhancing overall mood.

- **Increasing Focus and Mental Clarity:** Staying hydrated and eating anti-inflammatory foods can improve cognitive function, helping you feel clearer, more focused, and resilient.

This plan promotes a balanced approach to detox, connecting physical wellness with mental clarity and emotional resilience. It's a comprehensive way to support mind-body health in your cleansing journey!

Date: _____     Day of Cleanse:_____

## Morning Reflection

**How did I feel when I woke up today?**
*(Consider energy levels, mood, physical comfort)*

_____

_____

**Today's Intention** *(Set a positive intention or goal for today, such as "stay hydrated" or "practice patience")*

_____

_____

**Hydration Tracker** *(Check off each glass of water)*

☐ 1   ☐ 2   ☐ 3   ☐ 4   ☐ 5   ☐ 6   ☐ 7   ☐ 8

## Midday Check-In

**Energy & Mood:** *(Circle your current mood)*

😁 Happy | 😊 Calm | 😌 Content

😔 Tired | 😣 Stressed | 😰 Anxious

**Notes:** *(Briefly describe how you feel physically and mentally)*

_____

_____

**Mindful Eating Reflection:**
What did you enjoy about your meals so far?

_____

_____

How did you practice mindful eating today? (e.g., eating slowly, savoring flavors)

_____

_____

## Evening Reflection

**Dinner & Evening Tea:** *(How did today's meals and the Fuller Cleanze Tea make you feel?)*

_____

**Gratitude:** *(List three things you're grateful for today)*

1 _____

2 _____

3 _____

**Physical Movement:** *(What movement or exercise did you do today?)*

_____

**Sleep Preparation:** *(List any calming evening rituals, like stretching or meditation, that you practiced before bed)*

_____

_____

_____

## Overall Reflection

**Today's Highlight:** *(What was the best part of your day?)*

_____

**Any Challenges?** *(What did you find challenging, and how did you manage it?)*

_____

**Notes for Tomorrow:** *(Any thoughts or adjustments you'd like to make for tomorrow's cleanse journey)*

_____

# DAY 01

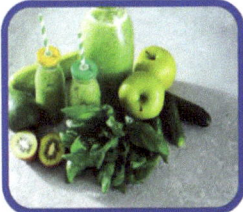

### Breakfast

Green smoothie made with spinach, kale, cucumber, apple, lemon juice, and a tablespoon of chia seeds.

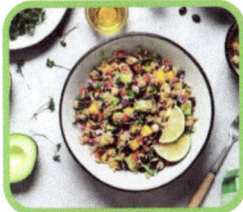

### Lunch

Quinoa salad with mixed vegetables, avocado, and a light lemon vinaigrette.

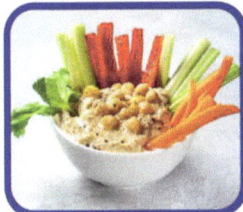

### Snack

Sliced bell peppers dipped in homemade hummus.

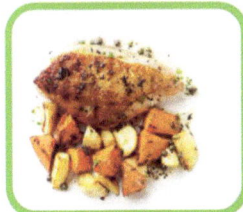

### Dinner

Baked salmon with steamed asparagus and a side of roasted sweet potatoes.

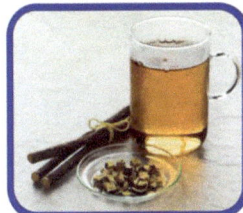

### Evening

Enjoy a cup of dandelion root tea.

Date: _____     Day of Cleanse: _____

## Morning Reflection

**How did I feel when I woke up today?**
*(Consider energy levels, mood, physical comfort)*

_____

_____

**Today's Intention** *(Set a positive intention or goal for today, such as "stay hydrated" or "practice patience")*

_____

_____

**Hydration Tracker** *(Check off each glass of water)*

☐ 1    ☐ 2    ☐ 3    ☐ 4    ☐ 5    ☐ 6    ☐ 7    ☐ 8

## Midday Check-In

**Energy & Mood:** *(Circle your current mood)*

😄 Happy | 😊 Calm | 😌 Content

😔 Tired | 😣 Stressed | 😨 Anxious

**Notes:** *(Briefly describe how you feel physically and mentally)*

_____

_____

**Mindful Eating Reflection:**
What did you enjoy about your meals so far?

_____

_____

How did you practice mindful eating today? (e.g., eating slowly, savoring flavors)

_____

_____

## Evening Reflection

**Dinner & Evening Tea:** *(How did today's meals and the Fuller Cleanze Tea make you feel?)*

_____

**Physical Movement:** *(What movement or exercise did you do today?)*

_____

**Gratitude:** *(List three things you're grateful for today)*

1 _____

2 _____

3 _____

**Sleep Preparation:** *(List any calming evening rituals, like stretching or meditation, that you practiced before bed)*

_____

_____

_____

## Overall Reflection

**Today's Highlight:** *(What was the best part of your day?)*

_____

**Any Challenges?** *(What did you find challenging, and how did you manage it?)*

_____

**Notes for Tomorrow:** *(Any thoughts or adjustments you'd like to make for tomorrow's cleanse journey)*

_____

# DAY 02

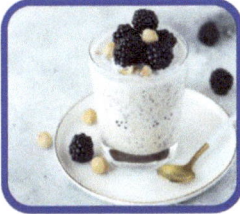

**Breakfast**

Overnight chia seed pudding made with almond milk, topped with berries and a sprinkle of flaxseeds.

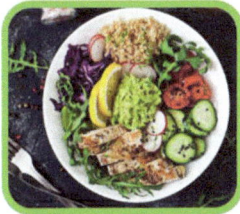

**Lunch**

Mixed green salad with grilled chicken, cherry tomatoes, cucumber, and a lemon-tahini dressing.

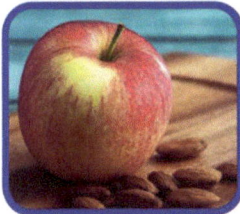

**Snack**

Almonds and a small apple.

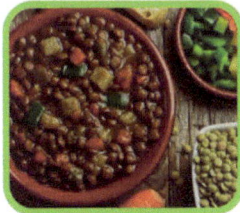

**Dinner**

Lentil soup with added vegetables like carrots, celery, and onions.

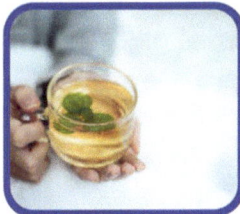

**Evening**

Sip on a cup of Fuller Cleanze Detox Tea.

Date: _____  Day of Cleanse: _____

## Morning Reflection

**How did I feel when I woke up today?**
*(Consider energy levels, mood, physical comfort)*

**Today's Intention** *(Set a positive intention or goal for today, such as "stay hydrated" or "practice patience")*

_____  _____

_____  _____

**Hydration Tracker** *(Check off each glass of water)*

☐ 1  ☐ 2  ☐ 3  ☐ 4  ☐ 5  ☐ 6  ☐ 7  ☐ 8

## Midday Check-In

**Energy & Mood:** *(Circle your current mood)*

😁 Happy | 😊 Calm | 😌 Content

😔 Tired | 😣 Stressed | 😰 Anxious

**Notes:** *(Briefly describe how you feel physically and mentally)*

_____

_____

**Mindful Eating Reflection:**
What did you enjoy about your meals so far?

_____

_____

How did you practice mindful eating today? *(e.g., eating slowly, savoring flavors)*

_____

_____

## Evening Reflection

**Dinner & Evening Tea:** *(How did today's meals and the Fuller Cleanze Tea make you feel?)*

_____

**Physical Movement:** *(What movement or exercise did you do today?)*

_____

**Gratitude:** *(List three things you're grateful for today)*

1 _____

2 _____

3 _____

**Sleep Preparation:** *(List any calming evening rituals, like stretching or meditation, that you practiced before bed)*

_____

## Overall Reflection

**Today's Highlight:** *(What was the best part of your day?)*

_____

**Any Challenges?** *(What did you find challenging, and how did you manage it?)*

_____

**Notes for Tomorrow:** *(Any thoughts or adjustments you'd like to make for tomorrow's cleanse journey)*

_____

# DAY 03

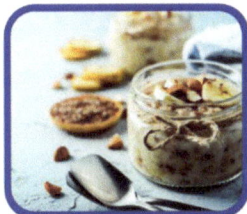

### Breakfast

Oatmeal topped with sliced bananas, walnuts, and a drizzle of honey.

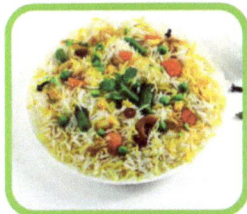

### Lunch

Brown rice bowl with sautéed mixed vegetables, tofu, and a soy-ginger dressing.

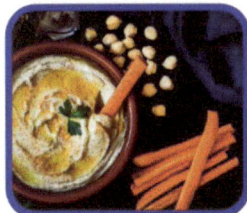

### Snack

Carrot sticks with almond butter.

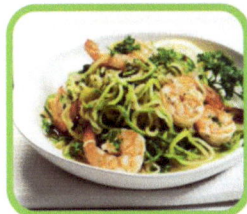

### Dinner

Grilled shrimp skewers with zucchini noodles and a homemade pesto sauce.

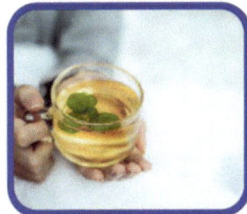

### Evening

Enjoy a cup of Fuller Cleanze Detox Tea.

Date: _____    Day of Cleanse:_____

## Morning Reflection

**How did I feel when I woke up today?**
*(Consider energy levels, mood, physical comfort)*

_____

_____

**Today's Intention** *(Set a positive intention or goal for today, such as "stay hydrated" or "practice patience")*

_____

_____

**Hydration Tracker** *(Check off each glass of water)*

☐ 1   ☐ 2   ☐ 3   ☐ 4   ☐ 5   ☐ 6   ☐ 7   ☐ 8

## Midday Check-In

**Energy & Mood:** *(Circle your current mood)*

😁 Happy | 🙂 Calm | 😊 Content

😔 Tired | 😣 Stressed | 😰 Anxious

**Notes:** *(Briefly describe how you feel physically and mentally)*

_____

_____

**Mindful Eating Reflection:**
What did you enjoy about your meals so far?

_____

_____

How did you practice mindful eating today? (e.g., eating slowly, savoring flavors)

_____

_____

## Evening Reflection

**Dinner & Evening Tea:** *(How did today's meals and the Fuller Cleanze Tea make you feel?)*

_____

**Gratitude:** *(List three things you're grateful for today)*

1 _____

2 _____

3 _____

**Physical Movement:** *(What movement or exercise did you do today?)*

_____

**Sleep Preparation:** *(List any calming evening rituals, like stretching or meditation, that you practiced before bed)*

_____

_____

## Overall Reflection

**Today's Highlight:** *(What was the best part of your day?)*

_____

**Any Challenges?** *(What did you find challenging, and how did you manage it?)*

_____

**Notes for Tomorrow:** *(Any thoughts or adjustments you'd like to make for tomorrow's cleanse journey)*

_____

# DAY 04

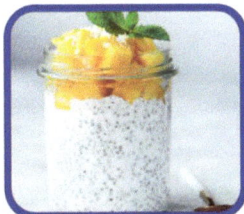

### Breakfast
Smoothie with mango, spinach, coconut water, and a scoop of chia seeds.

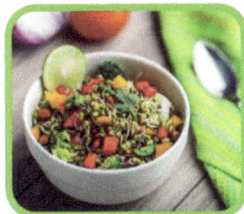

### Lunch
Lentil salad with arugula, cucumber, diced red pepper, and a lemon-olive oil dressing.

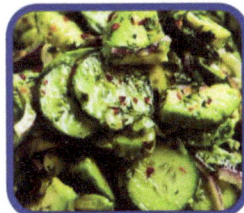

### Snack
Sliced cucumber with guacamole.

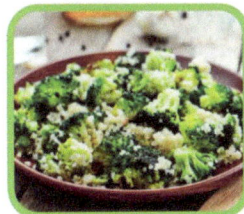

### Dinner
Baked cod with a side of quinoa and steamed broccoli.

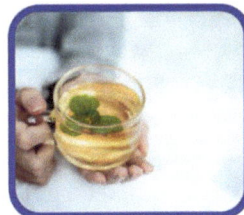

### Evening
Fuller Cleanze Detox Tea.

Date: _____ Day of Cleanse: _____

## Morning Reflection

**How did I feel when I woke up today?**
*(Consider energy levels, mood, physical comfort)*

_____

_____

**Today's Intention** *(Set a positive intention or goal for today, such as "stay hydrated" or "practice patience")*

_____

**Hydration Tracker** *(Check off each glass of water)*

☐ 1  ☐ 2  ☐ 3  ☐ 4  ☐ 5  ☐ 6  ☐ 7  ☐ 8

## Midday Check-In

**Energy & Mood:** *(Circle your current mood)*

😁 Happy | 😊 Calm | 😌 Content

😔 Tired | 😤 Stressed | 😰 Anxious

**Notes:** *(Briefly describe how you feel physically and mentally)*

_____

_____

**Mindful Eating Reflection:**
What did you enjoy about your meals so far?

_____

How did you practice mindful eating today? (e.g., eating slowly, savoring flavors)

_____

_____

## Evening Reflection

**Dinner & Evening Tea:** *(How did today's meals and the Fuller Cleanze Tea make you feel?)*

_____

**Gratitude:** *(List three things you're grateful for today)*

1 _____

2 _____

3 _____

**Physical Movement:** *(What movement or exercise did you do today?)*

_____

**Sleep Preparation:** *(List any calming evening rituals, like stretching or meditation, that you practiced before bed)*

_____

## Overall Reflection

**Today's Highlight:** *(What was the best part of your day?)*

_____

**Any Challenges?** *(What did you find challenging, and how did you manage it?)*

_____

**Notes for Tomorrow:** *(Any thoughts or adjustments you'd like to make for tomorrow's cleanse journey)*

_____

# DAY 05

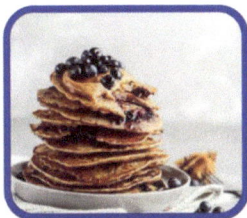

### Breakfast

Buckwheat pancakes topped with blueberries and a touch of almond butter.

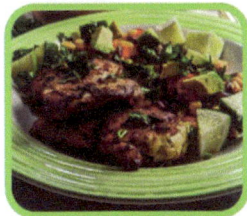

### Lunch

Sweet potato and black bean salad with avocado, cherry tomatoes, and a cilantro-lime dressing.

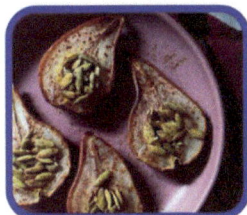

### Snack

A handful of pumpkin seeds and a small pear.

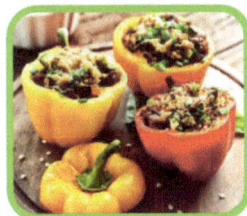

### Dinner

Stuffed bell peppers with a mixture of ground turkey, vegetables, and brown rice.

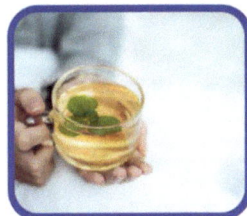

### Evening

Relax with Fuller Cleanze Detox Tea.

Date: _____  Day of Cleanse: _____

## Morning Reflection

**How did I feel when I woke up today?**
*(Consider energy levels, mood, physical comfort)*

_____

_____

**Today's Intention** *(Set a positive intention or goal for today, such as "stay hydrated" or "practice patience")*

_____

_____

**Hydration Tracker** *(Check off each glass of water)*

☐ 1   ☐ 2   ☐ 3   ☐ 4   ☐ 5   ☐ 6   ☐ 7   ☐ 8

## Midday Check-In

**Energy & Mood:** *(Circle your current mood)*

😄 Happy | 🙂 Calm | 😌 Content

😔 Tired | 😣 Stressed | 😰 Anxious

**Notes:** *(Briefly describe how you feel physically and mentally)*

_____

_____

**Mindful Eating Reflection:**
What did you enjoy about your meals so far?

_____

_____

How did you practice mindful eating today? (e.g., eating slowly, savoring flavors)

_____

_____

## Evening Reflection

**Dinner & Evening Tea:** *(How did today's meals and the Fuller Cleanze Tea make you feel?)*

_____

**Gratitude:** *(List three things you're grateful for today)*

1 _____

2 _____

3 _____

**Physical Movement:** *(What movement or exercise did you do today?)*

_____

**Sleep Preparation:** *(List any calming evening rituals, like stretching or meditation, that you practiced before bed)*

_____

_____

## Overall Reflection

**Today's Highlight:** *(What was the best part of your day?)*

_____

**Any Challenges?** *(What did you find challenging, and how did you manage it?)*

_____

**Notes for Tomorrow:** *(Any thoughts or adjustments you'd like to make for tomorrow's cleanse journey)*

_____

# DAY 06

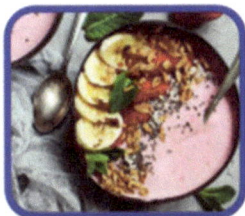

### Breakfast

Smoothie bowl with blended bananas, strawberries, and almond milk topped with granola.

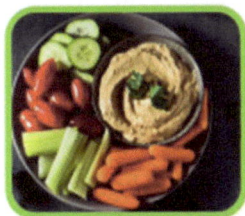

### Lunch

Grilled veggie wrap with hummus, bell peppers, spinach, and cucumbers.

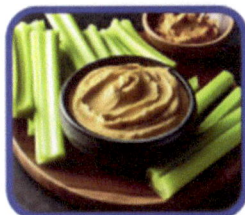

### Snack

Celery sticks with a light almond butter dip.

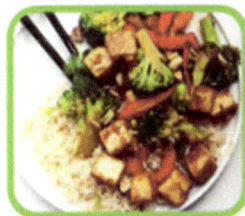

### Dinner

Vegetable stir-fry with tofu, broccoli, snap peas, and carrots over brown rice.

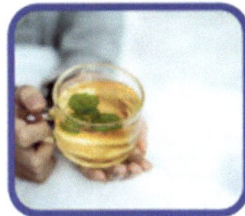

### Evening

Fuller Cleanze Detox Tea

Date: _____  Day of Cleanse: _____

## Morning Reflection

**How did I feel when I woke up today?**
*(Consider energy levels, mood, physical comfort)*

_____

_____

**Today's Intention** *(Set a positive intention or goal for today, such as "stay hydrated" or "practice patience")*

_____

_____

**Hydration Tracker** *(Check off each glass of water)*

☐ 1   ☐ 2   ☐ 3   ☐ 4   ☐ 5   ☐ 6   ☐ 7   ☐ 8

## Midday Check-In

**Energy & Mood:** *(Circle your current mood)*

😬 Happy | 😊 Calm | 😌 Content

😫 Tired | 😣 Stressed | 😰 Anxious

**Notes:** *(Briefly describe how you feel physically and mentally)*

_____

_____

_____

**Mindful Eating Reflection:**
What did you enjoy about your meals so far?

_____

_____

How did you practice mindful eating today? (e.g., eating slowly, savoring flavors)

_____

_____

## Evening Reflection

**Dinner & Evening Tea:** *(How did today's meals and the Fuller Cleanze Tea make you feel?)*

_____

**Gratitude:** *(List three things you're grateful for today)*

1 _____

2 _____

3 _____

**Physical Movement:** *(What movement or exercise did you do today?)*

_____

**Sleep Preparation:** *(List any calming evening rituals, like stretching or meditation, that you practiced before bed)*

_____

_____

## Overall Reflection

**Today's Highlight:** *(What was the best part of your day?)*

_____

**Any Challenges?** *(What did you find challenging, and how did you manage it?)*

_____

**Notes for Tomorrow:** *(Any thoughts or adjustments you'd like to make for tomorrow's cleanse journey)*

_____

# DAY 07

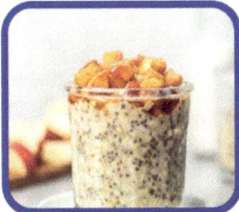

### Breakfast

Oats soaked overnight with almond milk, chia seeds, and a sprinkle of cinnamon, topped with apple slices.

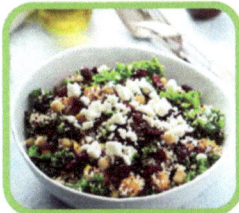

### Lunch

Chickpea and kale salad with a tahini dressing.

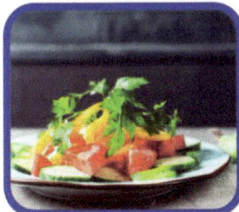

### Snack

Sliced bell peppers and cucumber with salsa.

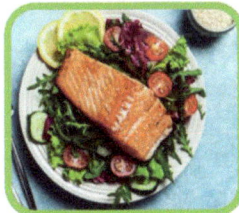

### Dinner

Grilled salmon with a mixed greens salad and a side of roasted beet slices.

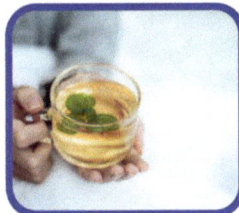

### Evening

Fuller Cleanze Detox Tea

Date: _____  Day of Cleanse: _____

## Morning Reflection

**How did I feel when I woke up today?**
*(Consider energy levels, mood, physical comfort)*

**Today's Intention** *(Set a positive intention or goal for today, such as "stay hydrated" or "practice patience")*

_____  _____

_____  _____

**Hydration Tracker** *(Check off each glass of water)*

☐ 1  ☐ 2  ☐ 3  ☐ 4  ☐ 5  ☐ 6  ☐ 7  ☐ 8

## Midday Check-In

**Energy & Mood:** *(Circle your current mood)*

😄 Happy | 😊 Calm | 😌 Content

😔 Tired | 😣 Stressed | 😰 Anxious

**Notes:** *(Briefly describe how you feel physically and mentally)*

**Mindful Eating Reflection:**
What did you enjoy about your meals so far?

_____

_____

How did you practice mindful eating today?
(e.g., eating slowly, savoring flavors)

_____

_____

## Evening Reflection

**Dinner & Evening Tea:** *(How did today's meals and the Fuller Cleanze Tea make you feel?)*

_____

**Physical Movement:** *(What movement or exercise did you do today?)*

_____

**Gratitude:** *(List three things you're grateful for today)*

1 _____

2 _____

3 _____

**Sleep Preparation:** *(List any calming evening rituals, like stretching or meditation, that you practiced before bed)*

## Overall Reflection

**Today's Highlight:** *(What was the best part of your day?)*

_____

**Any Challenges?** *(What did you find challenging, and how did you manage it?)*

_____

**Notes for Tomorrow:** *(Any thoughts or adjustments you'd like to make for tomorrow's cleanse journey)*

_____

# DAY 08

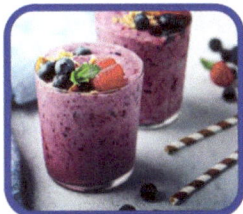

### Breakfast

Smoothie with mixed berries, a handful of spinach, a slice of ginger, and coconut water.

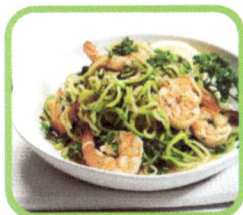

### Lunch

Zucchini noodles tossed with pesto, cherry tomatoes, and grilled shrimp.

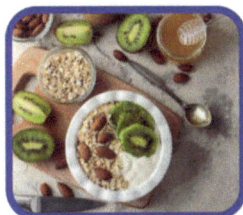

### Snack

Handful of almonds and a few slices of kiwi.

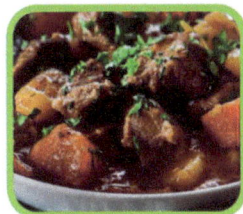

### Dinner

Lentil stew with carrots, celery, tomatoes, and fresh herbs.

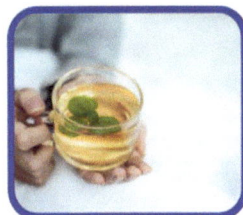

### Evening

Fuller Cleanze Detox Tea

Date: _____    Day of Cleanse: _____

## Morning Reflection

**How did I feel when I woke up today?**
*(Consider energy levels, mood, physical comfort)*

_____

_____

**Today's Intention** *(Set a positive intention or goal for today, such as "stay hydrated" or "practice patience")*

_____

**Hydration Tracker** *(Check off each glass of water)*

☐ 1  ☐ 2  ☐ 3  ☐ 4  ☐ 5  ☐ 6  ☐ 7  ☐ 8

## Midday Check-In

**Energy & Mood:** *(Circle your current mood)*

😄 Happy | 🙂 Calm | 😌 Content

😔 Tired | 😖 Stressed | 😰 Anxious

**Notes:** *(Briefly describe how you feel physically and mentally)*

_____

_____

**Mindful Eating Reflection:**
What did you enjoy about your meals so far?

_____

_____

How did you practice mindful eating today? (e.g., eating slowly, savoring flavors)

_____

_____

## Evening Reflection

**Dinner & Evening Tea:** *(How did today's meals and the Fuller Cleanze Tea make you feel?)*

_____

**Physical Movement:** *(What movement or exercise did you do today?)*

_____

**Gratitude:** *(List three things you're grateful for today)*

1 _____

2 _____

3 _____

**Sleep Preparation:** *(List any calming evening rituals, like stretching or meditation, that you practiced before bed)*

_____

_____

## Overall Reflection

**Today's Highlight:** *(What was the best part of your day?)*

_____

**Any Challenges?** *(What did you find challenging, and how did you manage it?)*

_____

**Notes for Tomorrow:** *(Any thoughts or adjustments you'd like to make for tomorrow's cleanse journey)*

_____

# DAY 09

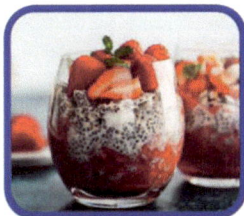

**Breakfast**

Greek yogurt with chia seeds, a few sliced strawberries, and a sprinkle of walnuts.

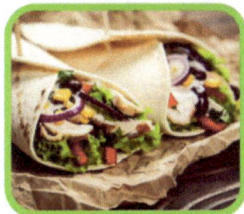

**Lunch**

Veggie wrap with a whole grain tortilla, mixed greens, shredded carrots, avocado, and a light tahini drizzle.

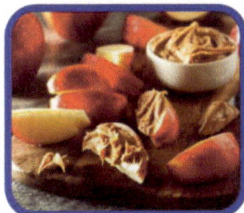

**Snack**

Sliced apple with almond butter.

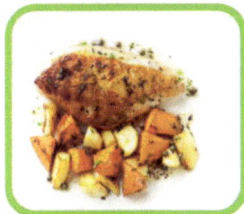

**Dinner**

Baked chicken breast with a side of steamed green beans and roasted sweet potatoes.

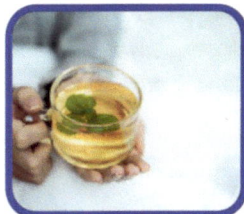

**Evening**

Fuller Cleanze Detox Tea

Date:_____ Day of Cleanse:_____

## Morning Reflection

**How did I feel when I woke up today?**
*(Consider energy levels, mood, physical comfort)*

_____

_____

**Today's Intention** *(Set a positive intention or goal for today, such as "stay hydrated" or "practice patience")*

_____

_____

**Hydration Tracker** *(Check off each glass of water)*

☐ 1  ☐ 2  ☐ 3  ☐ 4  ☐ 5  ☐ 6  ☐ 7  ☐ 8

## Midday Check-In

**Energy & Mood:** *(Circle your current mood)*

😆 Happy | 🙂 Calm | 😌 Content

😔 Tired | 😣 Stressed | 😰 Anxious

**Notes:** *(Briefly describe how you feel physically and mentally)*

_____

_____

**Mindful Eating Reflection:**
What did you enjoy about your meals so far?

_____

_____

How did you practice mindful eating today?
(e.g., eating slowly, savoring flavors)

_____

_____

## Evening Reflection

**Dinner & Evening Tea:** *(How did today's meals and the Fuller Cleanze Tea make you feel?)*

_____

**Gratitude:** *(List three things you're grateful for today)*

1 _____

2 _____

3 _____

**Physical Movement:** *(What movement or exercise did you do today?)*

_____

**Sleep Preparation:** *(List any calming evening rituals, like stretching or meditation, that you practiced before bed)*

_____

_____

## Overall Reflection

**Today's Highlight:** *(What was the best part of your day?)*

_____

**Any Challenges?** *(What did you find challenging, and how did you manage it?)*

_____

**Notes for Tomorrow:** *(Any thoughts or adjustments you'd like to make for tomorrow's cleanse journey)*

_____

# DAY 10

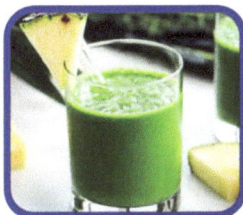

### Breakfast

Smoothie with kale, pineapple, cucumber, a slice of ginger, and coconut water.

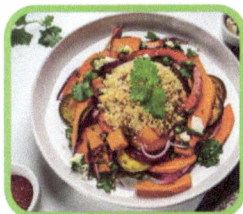

### Lunch

Warm quinoa bowl with roasted vegetables (bell peppers, zucchini, and carrots) and a drizzle of tahini dressing.

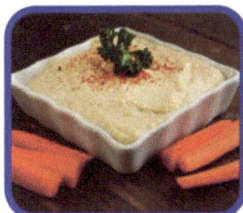

### Snack

Sliced carrots and celery with a light hummus dip.

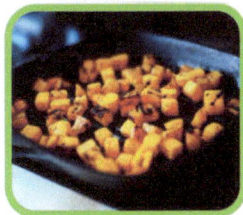

### Dinner

Baked halibut with a side of steamed asparagus and roasted butternut squash.

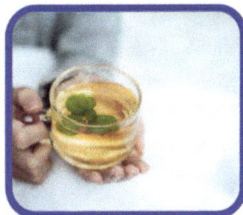

### Evening

Fuller Cleanze Detox Tea

Date: _____  Day of Cleanse: _____

## Morning Reflection

**How did I feel when I woke up today?**
*(Consider energy levels, mood, physical comfort)*

_____

_____

**Today's Intention** *(Set a positive intention or goal for today, such as "stay hydrated" or "practice patience")*

_____

_____

**Hydration Tracker** *(Check off each glass of water)*

☐ 1  ☐ 2  ☐ 3  ☐ 4  ☐ 5  ☐ 6  ☐ 7  ☐ 8

## Midday Check-In

**Energy & Mood:** *(Circle your current mood)*

😁 Happy | 😊 Calm | 😌 Content

😔 Tired | 😣 Stressed | 😰 Anxious

**Notes:** *(Briefly describe how you feel physically and mentally)*

_____

_____

**Mindful Eating Reflection:**
What did you enjoy about your meals so far?

_____

_____

How did you practice mindful eating today? *(e.g., eating slowly, savoring flavors)*

_____

_____

## Evening Reflection

**Dinner & Evening Tea:** *(How did today's meals and the Fuller Cleanze Tea make you feel?)*

_____

**Physical Movement:** *(What movement or exercise did you do today?)*

_____

**Gratitude:** *(List three things you're grateful for today)*

1 _____

2 _____

3 _____

**Sleep Preparation:** *(List any calming evening rituals, like stretching or meditation, that you practiced before bed)*

_____

_____

## Overall Reflection

**Today's Highlight:** *(What was the best part of your day?)*

_____

**Any Challenges?** *(What did you find challenging, and how did you manage it?)*

_____

**Notes for Tomorrow:** *(Any thoughts or adjustments you'd like to make for tomorrow's cleanse journey)*

_____

# DAY 11

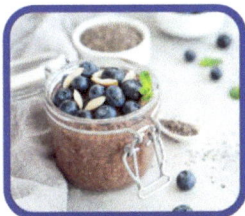

### Breakfast

Chia seed pudding with almond milk, topped with blueberries, almonds, and a dash of cinnamon.

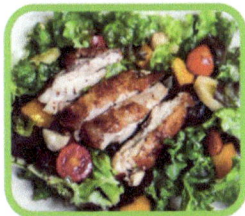

### Lunch

Mixed green salad with grilled chicken, avocado, cherry tomatoes, and a lemon-olive oil dressing.

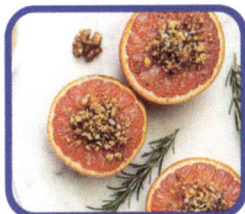

### Snack

A handful of walnuts and half a grapefruit.

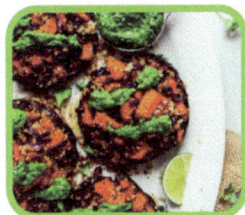

### Dinner

Stuffed portobello mushrooms with spinach, tomatoes, and quinoa.

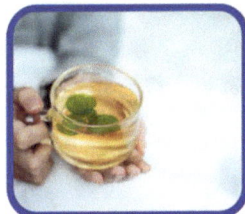

### Evening

Fuller Cleanze Detox Tea

Date: _____     Day of Cleanse:_____

## Morning Reflection

**How did I feel when I woke up today?**
*(Consider energy levels, mood, physical comfort)*

_____

_____

**Today's Intention** *(Set a positive intention or goal for today, such as "stay hydrated" or "practice patience")*

_____

_____

**Hydration Tracker** *(Check off each glass of water)*

☐ 1   ☐ 2   ☐ 3   ☐ 4   ☐ 5   ☐ 6   ☐ 7   ☐ 8

## Midday Check-In

**Energy & Mood:** *(Circle your current mood)*

😁 Happy | 😊 Calm | 😌 Content

😔 Tired | 😠 Stressed | 😰 Anxious

**Notes:** *(Briefly describe how you feel physically and mentally)*

_____

_____

**Mindful Eating Reflection:**
What did you enjoy about your meals so far?

_____

_____

How did you practice mindful eating today? *(e.g., eating slowly, savoring flavors)*

_____

_____

## Evening Reflection

**Dinner & Evening Tea:** *(How did today's meals and the Fuller Cleanze Tea make you feel?)*

_____

**Gratitude:** *(List three things you're grateful for today)*

1 _____

2 _____

3 _____

**Physical Movement:** *(What movement or exercise did you do today?)*

_____

**Sleep Preparation:** *(List any calming evening rituals, like stretching or meditation, that you practiced before bed)*

_____

## Overall Reflection

**Today's Highlight:** *(What was the best part of your day?)*

_____

**Any Challenges?** *(What did you find challenging, and how did you manage it?)*

_____

**Notes for Tomorrow:** *(Any thoughts or adjustments you'd like to make for tomorrow's cleanse journey)*

_____

# DAY 12

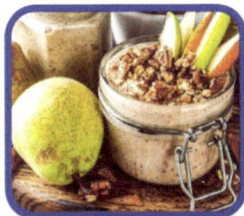

### Breakfast

Oatmeal with sliced pear, chia seeds, and a sprinkle of cinnamon.

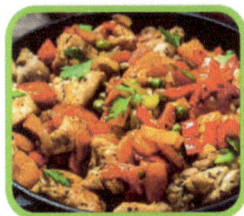

### Lunch

Chickpea and vegetable stir-fry with brown rice and a dash of turmeric.

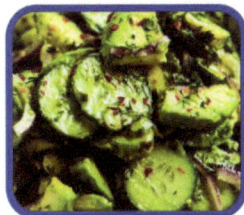

### Snack

Sliced cucumber with mashed avocado and a pinch of sea salt.

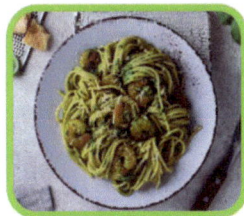

### Dinner

Zucchini noodles with grilled shrimp and a basil pesto sauce.

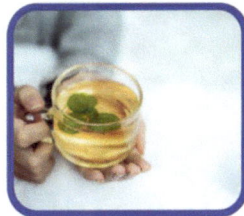

### Evening

Fuller Cleanze Detox Tea

Date:_____     Day of Cleanse:_____

## Morning Reflection

**How did I feel when I woke up today?**
*(Consider energy levels, mood, physical comfort)*

_____

_____

**Today's Intention** *(Set a positive intention or goal for today, such as "stay hydrated" or "practice patience")*

_____

_____

**Hydration Tracker** *(Check off each glass of water)*

☐ 1   ☐ 2   ☐ 3   ☐ 4   ☐ 5   ☐ 6   ☐ 7   ☐ 8

## Midday Check-In

**Energy & Mood:** *(Circle your current mood)*

😄 Happy | 😊 Calm | 😌 Content

😔 Tired | 😤 Stressed | 😰 Anxious

**Notes:** *(Briefly describe how you feel physically and mentally)*

_____

_____

**Mindful Eating Reflection:**
What did you enjoy about your meals so far?

_____

_____

How did you practice mindful eating today? *(e.g., eating slowly, savoring flavors)*

_____

_____

## Evening Reflection

**Dinner & Evening Tea:** *(How did today's meals and the Fuller Cleanze Tea make you feel?)*

_____

**Physical Movement:** *(What movement or exercise did you do today?)*

_____

**Gratitude:** *(List three things you're grateful for today)*

1 _____

2 _____

3 _____

**Sleep Preparation:** *(List any calming evening rituals, like stretching or meditation, that you practiced before bed)*

_____

_____

## Overall Reflection

**Today's Highlight:** *(What was the best part of your day?)*

_____

**Any Challenges?** *(What did you find challenging, and how did you manage it?)*

_____

**Notes for Tomorrow:** *(Any thoughts or adjustments you'd like to make for tomorrow's cleanse journey)*

_____

# DAY 13

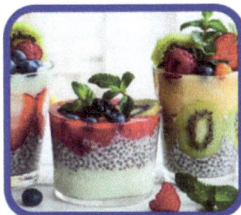

### Breakfast

Smoothie with strawberries, spinach, a tablespoon of chia seeds, and coconut water.

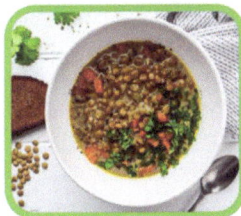

### Lunch

Lentil and vegetable soup with carrots, celery, and chopped greens.

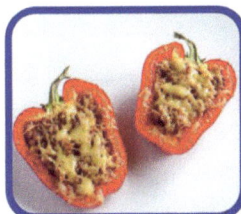

### Snack

Sliced bell peppers with homemade guacamole.

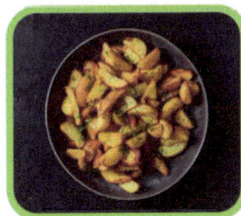

### Dinner

Grilled salmon with roasted Brussels sprouts and a side of sweet potato wedges.

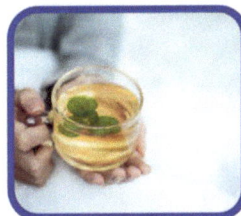

### Evening

Fuller Cleanze Detox Tea

Date: _____    Day of Cleanse: _____

## Morning Reflection

**How did I feel when I woke up today?**
*(Consider energy levels, mood, physical comfort)*

_____

_____

**Today's Intention** *(Set a positive intention or goal for today, such as "stay hydrated" or "practice patience")*

_____

**Hydration Tracker** *(Check off each glass of water)*

☐ 1   ☐ 2   ☐ 3   ☐ 4   ☐ 5   ☐ 6   ☐ 7   ☐ 8

## Midday Check-In

**Energy & Mood:** *(Circle your current mood)*

😁 Happy | 😊 Calm | 😌 Content

😔 Tired | 😣 Stressed | 😰 Anxious

**Notes:** *(Briefly describe how you feel physically and mentally)*

_____

_____

**Mindful Eating Reflection:**
What did you enjoy about your meals so far?

_____

_____

How did you practice mindful eating today? *(e.g., eating slowly, savoring flavors)*

_____

_____

## Evening Reflection

**Dinner & Evening Tea:** *(How did today's meals and the Fuller Cleanze Tea make you feel?)*

_____

**Physical Movement:** *(What movement or exercise did you do today?)*

_____

**Gratitude:** *(List three things you're grateful for today)*

1 _____

2 _____

3 _____

**Sleep Preparation:** *(List any calming evening rituals, like stretching or meditation, that you practiced before bed)*

_____

_____

## Overall Reflection

**Today's Highlight:** *(What was the best part of your day?)*

_____

**Any Challenges?** *(What did you find challenging, and how did you manage it?)*

_____

**Notes for Tomorrow:** *(Any thoughts or adjustments you'd like to make for tomorrow's cleanse journey)*

_____

# DAY 14

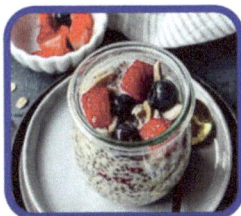

### Breakfast

Overnight oats with almond milk, chia seeds, and a topping of raspberries.

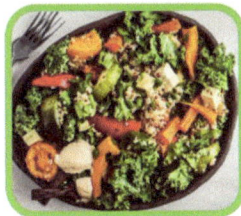

### Lunch

Quinoa salad with mixed greens, cucumber, cherry tomatoes, and a lemon-tahini dressing.

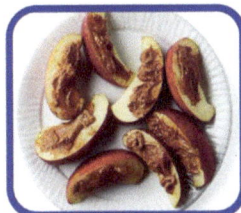

### Snack

Sliced apple with almond butter.

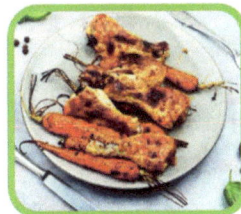

### Dinner

Baked chicken breast with a side of steamed green beans and roasted carrots.

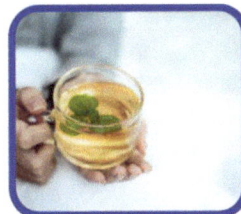

### Evening

Fuller Cleanze Detox Tea

Date: _____    Day of Cleanse: _____

## Morning Reflection

**How did I feel when I woke up today?**
*(Consider energy levels, mood, physical comfort)*

**Today's Intention** *(Set a positive intention or goal for today, such as "stay hydrated" or "practice patience")*

_____    _____

_____    _____

**Hydration Tracker** *(Check off each glass of water)*

☐ 1  ☐ 2  ☐ 3  ☐ 4  ☐ 5  ☐ 6  ☐ 7  ☐ 8

## Midday Check-In

**Energy & Mood:** *(Circle your current mood)*

😁 Happy | 😊 Calm | 😉 Content

😔 Tired | 😣 Stressed | 😰 Anxious

**Notes:** *(Briefly describe how you feel physically and mentally)*

_____

_____

**Mindful Eating Reflection:**
What did you enjoy about your meals so far?

_____

_____

How did you practice mindful eating today? *(e.g., eating slowly, savoring flavors)*

_____

_____

## Evening Reflection

**Dinner & Evening Tea:** *(How did today's meals and the Fuller Cleanze Tea make you feel?)*

_____

**Gratitude:** *(List three things you're grateful for today)*

1 _____

2 _____

3 _____

**Physical Movement:** *(What movement or exercise did you do today?)*

_____

**Sleep Preparation:** *(List any calming evening rituals, like stretching or meditation, that you practiced before bed)*

_____

_____

## Overall Reflection

**Today's Highlight:** *(What was the best part of your day?)*

_____

**Any Challenges?** *(What did you find challenging, and how did you manage it?)*

_____

**Notes for Tomorrow:** *(Any thoughts or adjustments you'd like to make for tomorrow's cleanse journey)*

_____

# DAY 15

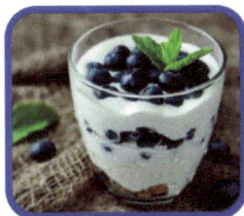

### Breakfast

Greek yogurt topped with blueberries, chia seeds, and a sprinkle of pumpkin seeds.

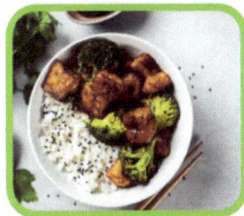

### Lunch

Brown rice bowl with sautéed mixed vegetables and tofu with a dash of coconut aminos.

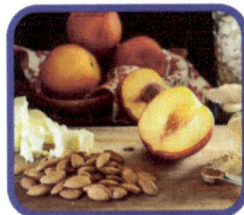

### Snack

A handful of almonds and a small peach.

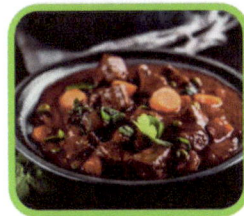

### Dinner

Lentil stew with carrots, celery, spinach, and herbs.

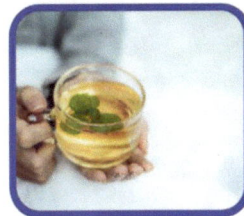

### Evening

Fuller Cleanze Detox Tea

Date: _____    Day of Cleanse: _____

## Morning Reflection

**How did I feel when I woke up today?**
*(Consider energy levels, mood, physical comfort)*

_____

_____

**Today's Intention** *(Set a positive intention or goal for today, such as "stay hydrated" or "practice patience")*

_____

_____

**Hydration Tracker** *(Check off each glass of water)*

☐ 1   ☐ 2   ☐ 3   ☐ 4   ☐ 5   ☐ 6   ☐ 7   ☐ 8

## Midday Check-In

**Energy & Mood:** *(Circle your current mood)*

😁 Happy | 😊 Calm | 😌 Content

😔 Tired | 😣 Stressed | 😰 Anxious

**Notes:** *(Briefly describe how you feel physically and mentally)*

_____

_____

**Mindful Eating Reflection:**
What did you enjoy about your meals so far?

_____

How did you practice mindful eating today? *(e.g., eating slowly, savoring flavors)*

_____

_____

## Evening Reflection

**Dinner & Evening Tea:** *(How did today's meals and the Fuller Cleanze Tea make you feel?)*

_____

**Gratitude:** *(List three things you're grateful for today)*

1 _____

2 _____

3 _____

**Physical Movement:** *(What movement or exercise did you do today?)*

_____

**Sleep Preparation:** *(List any calming evening rituals, like stretching or meditation, that you practiced before bed)*

_____

_____

## Overall Reflection

**Today's Highlight:** *(What was the best part of your day?)*

_____

**Any Challenges?** *(What did you find challenging, and how did you manage it?)*

_____

**Notes for Tomorrow:** *(Any thoughts or adjustments you'd like to make for tomorrow's cleanse journey)*

_____

# DAY 16

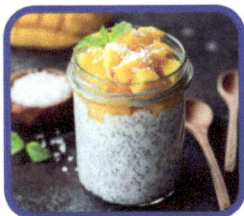

### Breakfast

Smoothie with mango, spinach, chia seeds, and coconut water.

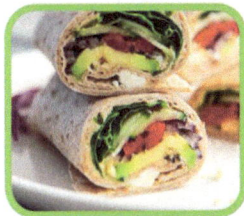

### Lunch

Roasted veggie wrap with hummus, bell peppers, cucumber, and greens in a whole grain tortilla.

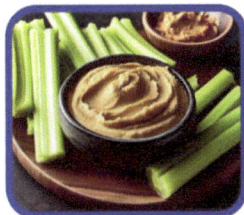

### Snack

Celery sticks with a light almond butter dip.

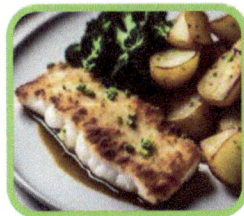

### Dinner

Baked cod with steamed broccoli and roasted sweet potatoes.

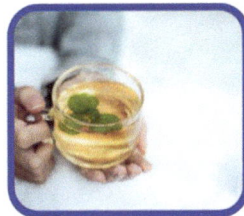

### Evening

Fuller Cleanze Detox Tea

Date: _____    Day of Cleanse: _____

## Morning Reflection

**How did I feel when I woke up today?**
*(Consider energy levels, mood, physical comfort)*

**Today's Intention** *(Set a positive intention or goal for today, such as "stay hydrated" or "practice patience")*

_____    _____

_____    _____

**Hydration Tracker** *(Check off each glass of water)*

☐ 1    ☐ 2    ☐ 3    ☐ 4    ☐ 5    ☐ 6    ☐ 7    ☐ 8

## Midday Check-In

**Energy & Mood:** *(Circle your current mood)*

😄 Happy | 😊 Calm | 😌 Content

😔 Tired | 😣 Stressed | 😰 Anxious

**Notes:** *(Briefly describe how you feel physically and mentally)*

_____

_____

**Mindful Eating Reflection:**
What did you enjoy about your meals so far?

_____

_____

How did you practice mindful eating today? *(e.g., eating slowly, savoring flavors)*

_____

_____

## Evening Reflection

**Dinner & Evening Tea:** *(How did today's meals and the Fuller Cleanze Tea make you feel?)*

_____

**Physical Movement:** *(What movement or exercise did you do today?)*

_____

**Gratitude:** *(List three things you're grateful for today)*

1 _____

2 _____

3 _____

**Sleep Preparation:** *(List any calming evening rituals, like stretching or meditation, that you practiced before bed)*

## Overall Reflection

**Today's Highlight:** *(What was the best part of your day?)*

_____

**Any Challenges?** *(What did you find challenging, and how did you manage it?)*

_____

**Notes for Tomorrow:** *(Any thoughts or adjustments you'd like to make for tomorrow's cleanse journey)*

_____

# DAY 17

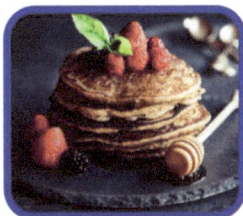

### Breakfast

Buckwheat pancakes with a few strawberries and a dash of almond butter.

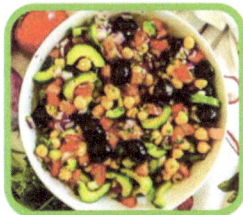

### Lunch

Mixed green salad with chickpeas, diced bell peppers, cucumbers, and a balsamic dressing.

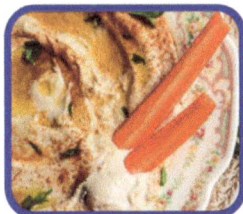

### Snack

Carrot sticks with homemade hummus.

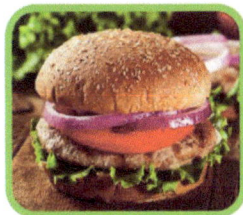

### Dinner

Grilled turkey burger wrapped in lettuce with a side of cucumber-tomato salad.

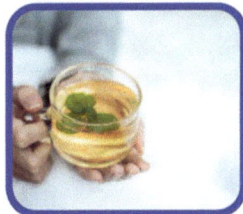

### Evening

Fuller Cleanze Detox Tea

Date:_____ Day of Cleanse:_____

## Morning Reflection

**How did I feel when I woke up today?**
*(Consider energy levels, mood, physical comfort)*

**Today's Intention** *(Set a positive intention or goal for today, such as "stay hydrated" or "practice patience")*

_____ _____

_____ _____

**Hydration Tracker** *(Check off each glass of water)*

☐ 1  ☐ 2  ☐ 3  ☐ 4  ☐ 5  ☐ 6  ☐ 7  ☐ 8

## Midday Check-In

**Energy & Mood:** *(Circle your current mood)*

😁 Happy | 😊 Calm | 😌 Content

😔 Tired | 😣 Stressed | 😰 Anxious

**Notes:** *(Briefly describe how you feel physically and mentally)*

_____

_____

**Mindful Eating Reflection:**
What did you enjoy about your meals so far?

_____

_____

How did you practice mindful eating today? *(e.g., eating slowly, savoring flavors)*

_____

_____

## Evening Reflection

**Dinner & Evening Tea:** *(How did today's meals and the Fuller Cleanze Tea make you feel?)*

_____

**Gratitude:** *(List three things you're grateful for today)*

1 _____

2 _____

3 _____

**Physical Movement:** *(What movement or exercise did you do today?)*

_____

**Sleep Preparation:** *(List any calming evening rituals, like stretching or meditation, that you practiced before bed)*

_____

## Overall Reflection

**Today's Highlight:** *(What was the best part of your day?)*

_____

**Any Challenges?** *(What did you find challenging, and how did you manage it?)*

_____

**Notes for Tomorrow:** *(Any thoughts or adjustments you'd like to make for tomorrow's cleanse journey)*

_____

# DAY 18

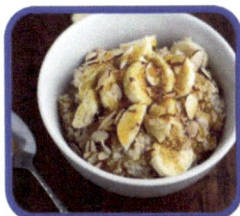

### Breakfast

Oatmeal with sliced banana, walnuts, and a pinch of cinnamon.

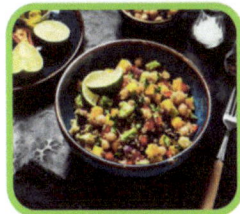

### Lunch

Brown rice and black bean salad with chopped greens, avocado, and lime juice.

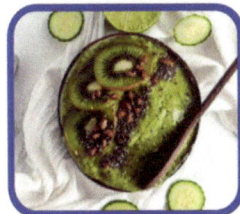

### Snack

A handful of pumpkin seeds and a few slices of kiwi.

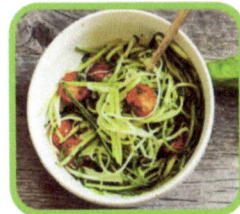

### Dinner

Grilled shrimp with zucchini noodles and a light tomato-basil sauce.

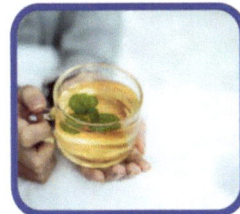

### Evening

Fuller Cleanze Detox Tea

Date: _____    Day of Cleanse: _____

## Morning Reflection

**How did I feel when I woke up today?**
*(Consider energy levels, mood, physical comfort)*

**Today's Intention** *(Set a positive intention or goal for today, such as "stay hydrated" or "practice patience")*

_____

_____

**Hydration Tracker** *(Check off each glass of water)*

☐ 1  ☐ 2  ☐ 3  ☐ 4  ☐ 5  ☐ 6  ☐ 7  ☐ 8

## Midday Check-In

**Energy & Mood:** *(Circle your current mood)*

😁 Happy | 😊 Calm | 😋 Content

😔 Tired | 😣 Stressed | 😰 Anxious

**Notes:** *(Briefly describe how you feel physically and mentally)*

**Mindful Eating Reflection:**
What did you enjoy about your meals so far?

_____

How did you practice mindful eating today? *(e.g., eating slowly, savoring flavors)*

## Evening Reflection

**Dinner & Evening Tea:** *(How did today's meals and the Fuller Cleanze Tea make you feel?)*

**Physical Movement:** *(What movement or exercise did you do today?)*

**Gratitude:** *(List three things you're grateful for today)*

1 _____

2 _____

3 _____

**Sleep Preparation:** *(List any calming evening rituals, like stretching or meditation, that you practiced before bed)*

_____

_____

## Overall Reflection

**Today's Highlight:** *(What was the best part of your day?)*

**Any Challenges?** *(What did you find challenging, and how did you manage it?)*

**Notes for Tomorrow:** *(Any thoughts or adjustments you'd like to make for tomorrow's cleanse journey)*

_____

# DAY 19

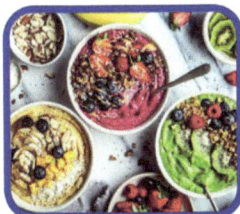

### Breakfast

Smoothie bowl with blended berries, spinach, and almond milk, topped with a sprinkle of flaxseeds.

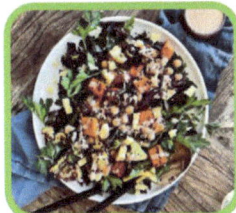

### Lunch

Quinoa salad with roasted beets, arugula, and a tahini-lemon dressing.

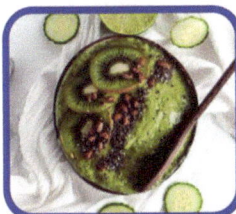

### Snack

Sliced bell peppers and cucumber with a yogurt dip.

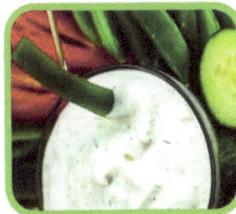

### Dinner

Grilled chicken breast with a side of steamed green beans and a roasted sweet potato.

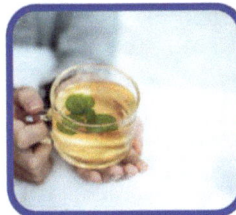

### Evening

Fuller Cleanze Detox Tea

Date: _____    Day of Cleanse: _____

## Morning Reflection

**How did I feel when I woke up today?**
*(Consider energy levels, mood, physical comfort)*

**Today's Intention** *(Set a positive intention or goal for today, such as "stay hydrated" or "practice patience")*

_____

_____

**Hydration Tracker** *(Check off each glass of water)*

☐ 1   ☐ 2   ☐ 3   ☐ 4   ☐ 5   ☐ 6   ☐ 7   ☐ 8

## Midday Check-In

**Energy & Mood:** *(Circle your current mood)*

😀 Happy | 😊 Calm | 😋 Content

😔 Tired | 😤 Stressed | 😰 Anxious

**Notes:** *(Briefly describe how you feel physically and mentally)*

**Mindful Eating Reflection:**
What did you enjoy about your meals so far?

_____

How did you practice mindful eating today? (e.g., eating slowly, savoring flavors)

_____

## Evening Reflection

**Dinner & Evening Tea:** *(How did today's meals and the Fuller Cleanze Tea make you feel?)*

**Physical Movement:** *(What movement or exercise did you do today?)*

**Gratitude:** *(List three things you're grateful for today)*

1 _____

2 _____

3 _____

**Sleep Preparation:** *(List any calming evening rituals, like stretching or meditation, that you practiced before bed)*

## Overall Reflection

**Today's Highlight:** *(What was the best part of your day?)*

**Any Challenges?** *(What did you find challenging, and how did you manage it?)*

**Notes for Tomorrow:** *(Any thoughts or adjustments you'd like to make for tomorrow's cleanse journey)*

_____

# DAY 20

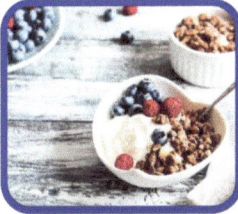

### Breakfast

Greek yogurt with chia seeds, fresh berries, and a dash of cinnamon.

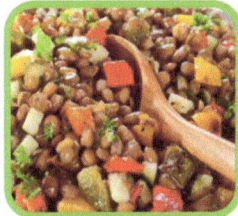

### Lunch

Roasted vegetable salad with lentils, mixed greens, and a balsamic dressing.

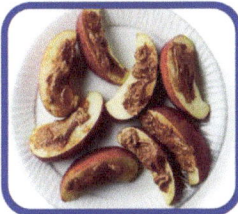

### Snack

A small apple with almond butter.

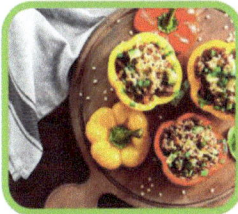

### Dinner

Stuffed bell peppers with quinoa, black beans, and vegetables.

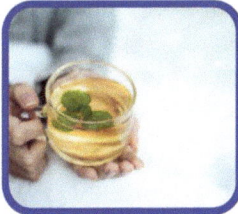

### Evening

Fuller Cleanze Detox Tea

Date: _____  Day of Cleanse: _____

## Morning Reflection

**How did I feel when I woke up today?**
*(Consider energy levels, mood, physical comfort)*

_____

_____

**Today's Intention** *(Set a positive intention or goal for today, such as "stay hydrated" or "practice patience")*

_____

**Hydration Tracker** *(Check off each glass of water)*

☐ 1  ☐ 2  ☐ 3  ☐ 4  ☐ 5  ☐ 6  ☐ 7  ☐ 8

## Midday Check-In

**Energy & Mood:** *(Circle your current mood)*

😁 Happy | 😊 Calm | 😌 Content

😔 Tired | 😣 Stressed | 😰 Anxious

**Notes:** *(Briefly describe how you feel physically and mentally)*

_____

_____

**Mindful Eating Reflection:**
What did you enjoy about your meals so far?

_____

_____

How did you practice mindful eating today? *(e.g., eating slowly, savoring flavors)*

_____

_____

## Evening Reflection

**Dinner & Evening Tea:** *(How did today's meals and the Fuller Cleanze Tea make you feel?)*

_____

**Gratitude:** *(List three things you're grateful for today)*

1 _____

2 _____

3 _____

**Physical Movement:** *(What movement or exercise did you do today?)*

_____

**Sleep Preparation:** *(List any calming evening rituals, like stretching or meditation, that you practiced before bed)*

_____

_____

## Overall Reflection

**Today's Highlight:** *(What was the best part of your day?)*

_____

**Any Challenges?** *(What did you find challenging, and how did you manage it?)*

_____

**Notes for Tomorrow:** *(Any thoughts or adjustments you'd like to make for tomorrow's cleanse journey)*

_____

# DAY 21

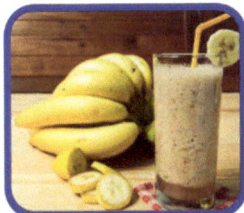

### Breakfast

Smoothie with banana, mixed berries, spinach, a slice of ginger, and almond milk.

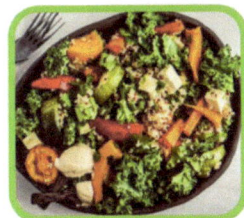

### Lunch

Chickpea and kale salad with cherry tomatoes, cucumber, and a lemon-tahini dressing.

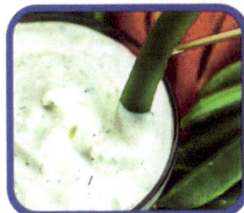

### Snack

Sliced cucumbers with guacamole.

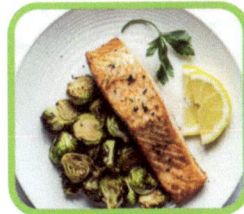

### Dinner

Baked salmon with roasted Brussels sprouts and mashed cauliflower.

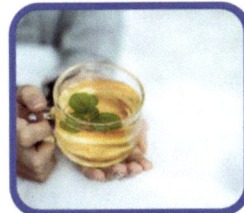

### Evening

Fuller Cleanze Detox Tea to conclude the cleanse.

# Final Tips for the Last Week of Your Cleanse

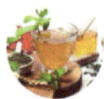

**Herbal Infusions:** For maximum effects, include your Fuller Cleanze Detox Tea every morning and before you go to bed.

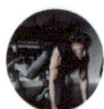

**Mindful Movement:** Aim for relaxing exercises like stretching, exercising and light Pilates to support circulation.

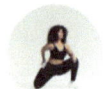

**Gentle Stretching:** Incorporate gentle stretching before bed to promote better sleep and relaxation.

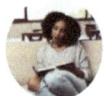

**Journaling:** Track how you feel each day—mentally and physically—throughout the cleanse. It can provide valuable insights for future wellness goals.

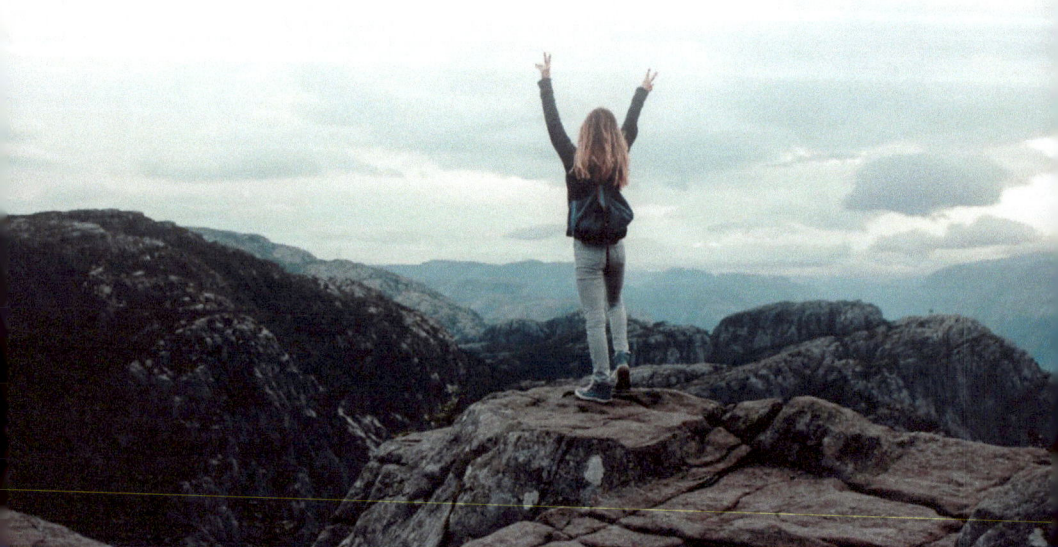

# Weekly Habits to Maintain Detox

- **Dry Brushing:** Stimulate circulation and promote skin detoxification with a soft dry brush before showering a few times a week.

- **Fuller Cleanze Detox Baths:** Relax in an Fuller Cleanze Detox salt bath for 20 minutes weekly to ease muscle tension and support detox.

- **Breathwork:** Incorporate deep-breathing exercises or meditation daily to reduce stress and enhance the body's natural detox processes.

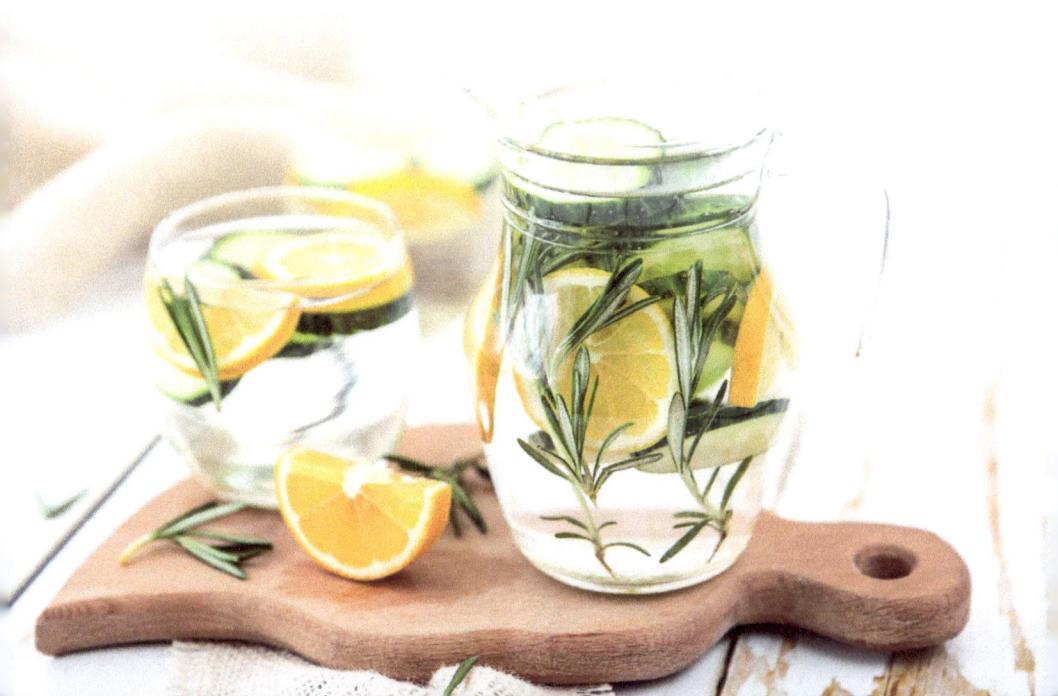

# Cleanse-Friendly Foods List

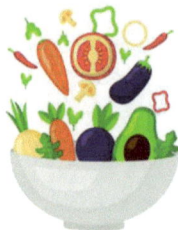

## MEATS & PROTEINS

*(Opt for organic, lean cuts and plant-based proteins)*

- **Fish:** Salmon, cod, trout, mackerel, sardines
- **Poultry:** Organic chicken breast, turkey breast
- **Plant-Based Proteins:** Lentils, chickpeas, black beans, quinoa, tofu, tempeh
- **Nuts & Seeds:** Almonds, walnuts, chia seeds, flaxseeds, pumpkin seeds (in moderation)
- **Eggs:** Organic, free-range eggs (for added protein)

## FRUITS

*(Aim for organic and low-sugar options)*

- **Berries:** Blueberries, strawberries, blackberries, raspberries
- **Citrus:** Lemon, lime, oranges, grapefruit
- **Apples and Pears**
- **Tropical Fruits (in moderation):** Pineapple, mango, papaya
- **Other Low-Sugar Options:** Avocado, kiwi, pomegranate, plums
- **Hydrating Fruits:** Watermelon, cucumber, cantaloupe

## VEGETABLES

*(Focus on leafy greens, cruciferous, and non-starchy veggies)*

- **Leafy Greens:** Spinach, kale, arugula, romaine, Swiss chard
- **Cruciferous Vegetables:** Broccoli, cauliflower, Brussels sprouts, cabbage
- **Roots & Tubers:** Sweet potatoes, beets, carrots, radishes
- **Alliums:** Garlic, onions, leeks, shallots
- **Other Vegetables:** Zucchini, bell peppers, asparagus, celery, cucumber, green beans, tomatoes
- **Herbs:** Parsley, cilantro, basil, mint

## WHOLE GRAINS

*(In moderation, ideally gluten-free and unprocessed)*

- Quinoa, brown rice, wild rice, millet, buckwheat, amaranth

## HEALTHY FATS

*(Include small amounts to support brain and hormone health)*

- **Oils:** Extra-virgin olive oil, coconut oil, avocado oil
- **Nuts & Seeds:** Almonds, walnuts, chia seeds, flaxseeds (use sparingly)
- **Avocado**

## DRINKS

*(Stay hydrated with these options while avoiding sugary beverages)*

- **Water:** Aim for 8-10 glasses daily
- **Herbal Teas:** Fuller Cleanze Detox Tea, dandelion root, chamomile, ginger, peppermint
- **Green Tea** (for an antioxidant boost)
- **Coconut Water** (unsweetened, for hydration)
- **Lemon or Lime Water:** Freshly squeezed for detox support
- **Smoothies:** Blend fruits, veggies, and plant-based milk for a hydrating snack

www.ingramcontent.com/pod-product-compliance
Lightning Source LLC
Chambersburg PA
CBHW040938030426
42335CB00001B/30